# Mental Health

## Understand How Our Culture is Making Us Sick

*(Exercises to Transform Negative Thoughts and Improve Well-being)*

**Rosella Block**

Published By **Phil Dawson**

# Rosella Block

All Rights Reserved

*Mental Health: Understand How Our Culture is Making Us Sick (Exercises to Transform Negative Thoughts and Improve Well-being)*

# ISBN 978-1-77485-912-4

No part of this guidebook shall be reproduced in any form without permission in writing from the publisher except in the case of brief quotations embodied in critical articles or reviews.

Legal & Disclaimer

The information contained in this ebook is not designed to replace or take the place of any form of medicine or professional medical advice. The information in this ebook has been provided for educational & entertainment purposes only.

The information contained in this book has been compiled from sources deemed reliable, and it is accurate to the best of the Author's knowledge; however, the Author cannot guarantee its accuracy and validity and cannot be held liable for any errors or omissions. Changes are periodically made to this book. You must consult your doctor or get professional medical advice before using any of the suggested remedies, techniques, or information in this book.

Upon using the information contained in this book, you agree to hold harmless the Author from and against any damages, costs, and expenses, including any legal fees potentially resulting from the application of any of the information provided by this guide. This disclaimer applies to any damages or injury caused by the use and application, whether directly or indirectly, of any advice or information presented, whether for breach of contract, tort, negligence, personal injury, criminal intent, or under any other cause of action.

You agree to accept all risks of using the information presented inside this book. You need to consult a professional medical practitioner in order to ensure you are both able and healthy enough to participate in this program.

## Table Of Contents

Chapter 1: How Important Is The Mental Health Topic............................... 1

Chapter 2: Covid-19 - The Effects Of Self Isolation On The Core Population .......... 25

Chapter 3: Students' Effects Of The Covid-19 Viral Virus.......................... 28

Chapter 4: The Relationship Between Mental Health, Happiness, Needs And Needs...................................... 65

Chapter 5: Self-Medication Is A Coping Tool...................................... 100

Chapter 6: The Pandemic And Its Dangers For Social Relations.............................. 108

Chapter 7: Find A Type Of Exercise That You Like ............................... 133

Chapter 8: Motivating People Surround You........................................ 148

Chapter 9: Attainable Goals .................. 167

# Chapter 1: How Important Is The Mental Health Topic

The current popularity of mental health advocacy has made it more urgent. Many foundations offer programs to raise awareness about mental health and emphasize that it should be taken seriously.

A growing awareness regarding mental health is important as each step men take exposes them to his holistic health concerns, including mental and physical health. Despite all the positives that technology has brought, there are many dangers. While technology and civilization are not to be demonized, it is possible to identify the drawbacks of technology and draw people's awareness. This is why awareness is crucial in this age.

What is Mental Health, exactly?

Mental health is a person's emotional and/or psychological well-being. It is used to evaluate a person's mental health by looking closely at their thought process to determine why they make certain decision. It also provides information about a person's ability to interact with others and how they behave when they are around them.

Our mental health can also include how well our brains adapt to and deal with everyday life's challenges and how well our ability to handle stress. These factors can have an impact on our choices.

In fact, poor mental well-being can impact physical health and the well-being the body. Persons with poor mental health might make dangerous decisions in their lives or suffer from severe heart disease.

Bad mental health can lead individuals to mental disorders. This can impact moods, thoughts, actions, and behavior. Mental disorders are so common that WHO believes that nearly half of all Americans will suffer from them at some point in their lives. Many people can become aware of their predisposing factors if they are educated. Others who are affected may seek treatment and can recover fully.

Many people suffer from mental conditions that have caused terrible illness, or aggravation of other underlying diseases. These conditions can cause severe harm, or even death. This is why it is so important to discuss mental illness, especially in cases where we might not be aware of potential mental health issues such as the COVID aftermath.

Mental health issues are not as common as physical problems that have symptoms right away. These issues tend to develop slowly and people might not be aware of their predisposition until they are already deeply affected. Slowly, behavioral patterns shift, social interaction decreases, and actions towards life issues change. This is a very mind-boggling topic.

Many people are affected by the COVID-19 Pandemic. They are suffering from mental illness, even if they do not know. The Centers for Disease Control reported that 40% of American adults struggle with mental health issues, or even substance abuse, three months after COVID-19 was declared a National Emergency. But, only 20% of American adults reported mental problems a year ago (2019). The sudden rise in these numbers is not an accident; the pandemic was a big factor.

## What is The Connection Between Mental Health & Social Relationships?

Humans are naturally social animals. They thrive on being in relationships for survival. The theory of evolution will reveal stories about how humans used to live in packs, hunt together, share food and do everything together. The communist system, where everybody worked together to pool resources and form a progressive community, was one of the most prominent forms of governance. Even though we have many different governance options today with less dependency on society and more individuality, the truth remains that we are social animals. We all identify with a group in some way socially. We don't want others to feel left out of our lives, whether they are family, friends, co-workers, or colleagues. Unfortunately, this story will not change.

People are more isolated today than they were in the past, making it necessary to be connected with others. It is true that our relationships are the most important parts of our human lives. People who have strong relationships with their family, friends, business partners, customers, or classmates, are more likely to be physically and mentally healthier.

Many people are in abusive relationships simply because they don't know anyone else. People would rather live with an abusive person, than with none. Although it is not true, being alone is better that being in a toxic partnership. People often find it easier to remain with relationships that don't make them feel appreciated. This is because they want the attention of someone, be it healthy or otherwise.

Psychological Medicine's 2014 research found that people who live together have a lower likelihood of suffering from mental illness, regardless how wealthy or poor they are.

Research shows that depression symptoms can be linked to loneliness, according to many researchers. Others have found that young adults will be less likely to engage in substance abuse if they are around people they care about. Many people who abuse drugs look for solace in these habits. People over 50 who feel overwhelmed by their lives would prefer to have a spouse/children to relate to. They can also have someone to check on their depression and offer support.

This shows how healthy relationships and strong social connections are crucial for both your mental and physical well-being.

Some of the benefits of regular social interaction include:

* Emotional well being

* Higher self-esteem

* Avoidance of anxiety, stress, and depression

* Empathy

* Reduces hypertension

* Improved immune system

* Longer life span

* Happiness

* Attractions

* Positive social feedback

Being alone and lacking social interaction can lead you to loneliness and other mental and physical health issues. You could also be lonely.

* It can cause disruptions in your sleep cycle. If you are alone, bored, or lonely, you will tend to fall asleep less often.

* Induce people to eat more, making them unhealthy and overweight.

* Increased risk of high bloodpressure, which can lead to fatal illnesses such as stroke, cancer, and cardiovascular disease.

* Increase body's levels of stress hormone cortisol

* Increase the likelihood of suffering mental diseases like dementia

For us to be healthy, it is essential that we have good health habits. For our mental and physical well-being, it is important to maintain good social relationships.

The importance of intimate relationships

Most people have at least one connection. It doesn't matter if they are working or not. All connections may not be intimate.

Intimate bonds are the relationships you have to your family, close friends, and those who really care about what you do. They have the ability to know your deepest secrets and most importantly, they can also see the ugly side of you. They have a relationship for goods reasons with you. Intimate connections, unlike business relationships, are not transactional. Instead they are deep and real.

Intimate relationships are important for people because they give them someone to talk to, someone they can trust, someone they can confide in.

Intimate relationships involve people who love and care deeply about you. A business partner can only keep you valuable if your business continues to make positive changes. However, any negative turn could cause the relationship to be irreparable. In other words, your closest relationships are the ones who will support and love you in your lowest points.

It is possible for people to make new friends. But these friends will only be of value if they become part or your intimate circle. To build close friendships with people, one must first understand their needs and then be able to communicate with them.

Our closest relationships are often in intimate environments like our home. Due to the level of intimacy, we spend a lot of time at the homes of our parents, spouses, close friends, and family. It is normal to be in intimate relationships with people, visit their parents' or friends' homes and discuss personal life issues.

You might wonder what happens if you are disconnected from the rest of the world. Your business associates will be unable to connect with you. You may feel alone and isolated. Such a situation must feel awful. This is the reality of what the entire world was faced with during the pandemic. People panicked so movement was restricted. Social distancing became mandatory, so people couldn't even see their family members.

Loneliness, while a valid concern, is not the only reason for poor mental health. Intimate relationships are essential for everyone. It's easy to let your spouse or sibling get a joke out of you. But it's much more fun if you can reminisce about your past experiences with your parents and siblings, or if you tell your friends about crazy things you did back then. According to Mental Health America's survey of Americans, 71% say they turn to their friends and family for help when stressed. Who can people turn to in times of social isolation and stress?

During the COVID-19 outbreak, internet interactions were strictly limited. It was difficult for co-workers to communicate electronically, while their families had to be in touch via email. Friends stayed connected via Facebook, Instagram, or other social media platforms. Multiple surveys have shown that online interactions don't feel as rewarding as those with physical contact. However, social media and technology are great tools for enhancing communication.

To give you an example, I could have deep, honest, heart-to–heart conversations with my friend in a physical setting. We could also hold hands, rub heads, and openly share our opinions without distractions. This makes the conversation feel real, and allows for seamless transitions between topics. Conversations over text can feel shallow because the other party may be messaging multiple people at the same time, or they might struggle to type long replies. This could lead to the conversation stalling.

Another reason physical communication can't be separated from online conversations is that cues are easily gotten through gestures, facial remarks and general body language. For example, I can sense if someone is pissed by their facial expression. I also can sense how emotionally invested they are in me.

The non-verbal communication cues account for more than half the communication in a physical setting. They are still there for obvious reasons. The facial expressions and body language can reveal many qualities, including guilt, passions, affections, dishonesty and many others. It is because of this that people love to talk about their problems with family and friends, their intimate relationships.

Many people became reliant on emails and texts to communicate with loved ones during the epidemic. It was easy to forget the genuine physical conversation which can be lost when we lose our ability to feel emotions in communication. Despite technology's advancements, it was difficult to communicate completely with loved ones during the Periods Of Isolation. This is when mental health problems began to appear, such as sadness, anxiety pressure and depression.

Psychological effects of social isolation

Studies show that prolonged periods of social isolation can have psychologically devastating effects on individuals. These psychological effects lead to increased mental health issues such as anxiety, fear and stress, as well as mental disorders like depression, anxiety and stress. This can cause young people to abuse substances, which could lead to other chronic conditions, such as diabetes, high blood sugar, cardiovascular diseases, cancer, and high blood pressure. These physiological effects increase the risk for dementia and schizophrenia among older adults. It's clear that the psychological effects of isolation on social life go well beyond mental health.

The feeling of happiness can be triggered by the physical connections with loved ones and friends. A happiness hormone (oxytocin), which is also secreted, is responsible for fostering happiness. What happens when social isolation and quarantine are mandatory?

When we consider prisoners in solitary confinement, with no human contact or relationship, it is easy to see this scenario. This lack in human contact and environmental awareness adversely impacts the prisoner's mental condition, leading to depression, permanent or semipermanent brain physiology or an existential crisis. This causes them to suffer from mental illnesses such as bipolarity, schizophrenia, major depressive disorder and dementia in extreme cases. Insanity and other significant functional impairments are often associated with these symptoms. Some people may eventually die.

Even though being in solitary confinement can be very different from being locked down or quarantine, the latter are less severe. There is still the possibility of communication, especially online. However, online communication is not a substitute for physical communication.

Many horse owners were kept in quarantine during the 2014 outbreak of equine Influenza. A large outbreak of the swine virus occurred in 2009 and many people were forced to remain isolated.

The symptoms of psychological stress were reported to be present in 34 percent of quarantined owners of horses. Only 12 percent of the general population showed similar symptoms. The swine virus caused symptoms in 28 percent of quarantined adult patients to show signs of traumatic mental disorders. This was compared with only 6% of the others.

Post-Traumatic Syndrome Disorder (PTSD), was also a prevalent condition among people after the lockdown was lifted. People feared going to public places, and they tried their best not to be in contact with others out of fear. Let's now discuss some of these psychological side effects.

* Distorted Sleeping Habits: This is when people don't leave the house and have trouble sleeping. Instead of getting 6-8

hours at night, they may get 3 or 4 hours each night with other naps during the day. As screen time increases, so do these sleeping disorders. This is because you are forced to communicate with family and friends through your computer and phone. The increased exposure to blue light from these devices can lead to insomnia and make it difficult for people to get to sleep. A healthy sleep routine is essential to maintain a healthy brain. Sleep disturbances have been shown to lead to stress, anxiety, and depression.

* Loneliness. This has been a growing epidemic since before the COVID crisis in 2020. According to Pew Research Center's 2018 survey, 10 percent of Americans feel alone all the time. There is no doubt that people feel isolated due to many factors. And the COVID pandemic only made matters worse.

Being alone is not only about having others around you, it's also about being able to make emotional connections with people. While you may feel lonely and depressed if there are many people around you, it is possible to be with one person and feel supported by the entire universe. Because there isn't much emotion to social media and the Internet, it doesn't help with loneliness. It's disconnected from the real world and people don't interact with each other. Most people have experienced loneliness at least once in their lives. If we have close friends and family, the loneliness is gone. However, chronic loneliness can lead to depression and anxiety.

* Post-Traumatic Syndrome Disorder (PTSD). Many people still have fears from past experiences. Consider a family member who was diagnosed by COVID. They eventually got better and got the

vaccine. In such cases, my subconscious may lean towards a fearful reaction to the relative's sneezing. This can make it difficult for the victim and could lead to the victim being afraid of being socially excluded if they become sick. This can slow down lead to depression, anxiety, or excessive levels of stress.

In addition to mental health issues, people can also suffer from physical issues from social isolation. Some examples are:

* Heart-Related Cardiovascular Diseases (or Cardiovascular Diseases): Human well-being depends on a variety of psychological, physiological, and biological factors. Numerous studies have shown that loneliness may increase the chance of developing a stroke, paralysis, heart disease, or any other cardiovascular disease by up to 30%.

People who lack support and communication from their loved ones turn to unhealthy behavior for comfort. This can increase stress levels, disrupt sleeping patterns and raise health risks.

* We have a poorer immune system. This prevents us easily getting infected by bacteria and disease-causing viruses. Studies show that people who are stressed and lonely tend to have more inflammation in their leukocytes. The immune system works by protecting the body from infections. Inflammation of the leukocytes (white cells) can cause the body to become less resilient. A weak immune system makes people vulnerable to infection and makes them more likely to be infected with bacteria or other disease-causing organisms. People who live alone are more likely than others to become sick.

It is clear from all that we have looked at that isolation can do more harm than good for our health holistically. Even though we all need our privacy, prolonged isolation poses serious risks to our physical and mental health.

## Chapter 2: Covid-19 - The Effects Of Self Isolation On The Core Population

The COVID-19 Pandemic was critical and required the control of the rapid spread of the coronavirus. The WHO and CDC led campaigns against social contact as coronavirus transmission was primarily airborne.

This pervasiveness is affecting nearly every aspect of human life: work, education. tourism. transportation. recreation.

Early 2020 was a time when we were able to run into old friends at the park. We exchanged pleasantries, had a handshake, or even a warm hug; but, the virus made these situations deadly and extra care was needed to have any physical contact. To prevent the spread, any physical contact with anyone was completely eliminated. Restaurants were closed and only delivery was allowed. Students could learn online without ever having to go to physical classes. Employees also started working remotely. No longer could people have the joy of telling jokes at lunch.

Many people, especially millennials, have neglected to notice the consequences of this isolation on the global productive population. This age group was predisposed towards loneliness, anxiety, depression and other mental health issues, both economically and socially. The pandemic made these mental health issues worse as more isolation became a normal part of daily life.

Let us examine how the effects on the core of humanity have been affected by the pandemic.

The majority population of the planet's millennials is composed of them. Statista states that the U.S. has a 22% generation of millennials, which is greater than any other generation.

The Millennials, 25- to 40-year-olds, are a large portion of the working class and largely comprise students. The Millennials make up the bulk of the world's productive population. It could spell doom for the whole world if the generation is not working hard enough.

## Chapter 3: Students' Effects of the COVID-19 Viral Virus

In order to stop the COVID-19 pandemic many international authorities closed schools at all grades, K-12 and college. Due to the effects of COVID-19, billions were affected at different levels. Therefore, it was necessary to find a way to support learners in keeping up with the curriculum. In order to protect every student's right to education, education policymakers and leaders in government developed other methods of instruction. Online learning was accepted by the majority of people until the gradual reopenings of schools and other learning institutions following vaccinations.

While online lessons may seem to have stopped, some activities have resumed to some degree; however, there are still many effects to be aware of, especially for those who are younger.

Virtual learning was the only option. However, the "solution" has brought about some issues that will have major implications for students' mental wellbeing.

* Depression as A Result of Classism. It's no secret that not all fingers can be equal. However, low-income families still work hard to obtain the best education. Many households cannot afford to live in an environment that has a fast internet connection in order to take an online class, especially during the current epidemic. Some homes lack the technology necessary to enable students to easily follow lectures online. The pandemic caused network providers to try and expand their reach, but rural areas have seen an increase in Internet demand as more people are staying at home and more networks are congested. Rural residents tend to be low-income.

They might not have sufficient money to purchase the required software and computers, or they may have a poor internet connection. The pandemic caused a drop in income, so high-income earners are able to provide for their children better than the socio-economically disadvantaged. This is a clear sign of a class gap, as the upper class can offer online learning structures to lower earners.

After the closure, schools were reopened. However, much of the curriculum was online. Teachers did not do any revisions. This made it more difficult for students with poor access to the internet to learn. They feel outcast and may start to drift towards depression. It doesn't end here; students who are privileged love to brag about and display their privileges, almost as though it's a game. Even though they might not be causing any harm, these effects subtly interfere with the sanity and interest of the underprivileged student. Instead they are more concerned with their social status. This causes them to be depressed, and it negatively impacts their mental health.

* Slower Learning: A psychological effect. Students gain less knowledge due to the imprudent nature of virtual learning and lockdowns. Teachers can feel the atmosphere in the classroom better to assess how well students absorb information, whether students seem confused or if they need to repeat certain lectures. It's especially common in practical courses where interaction is essential. But, the pandemic has forced them to limit their learning to online processes. This makes the interaction process more complicated and takes longer, much to the dismay of those who

are learning. This hinders students' ability to learn new information and causes them to lose enthusiasm. This is why these students don't want to wait until the end of the lesson and just go to "classes".

Even more alarming is the fact that these effects continue long after the pandemic. Motivation to learn and the desire to learn continue to be low. It would take a lot to rekindle that interest. The problem gets worse when the teacher attempts to refer to lessons learned during the pandemic. Most of these students were unable or unwillingly to absorb the information.

* Loneliness. School is fun because students can learn from others and have social interactions. Students look forward football, basketball, and other sporting events. Extra-curricular activities include

drama, school dance, opera, and many other exciting things. Education specialists have incorporated extra-curricular activities to ensure healthy distractions for students. "All work and no play makes Jack boring," so the educational curriculum includes fun activities that keep students entertained and happy. Learning becomes easier when students are happy.

Online learning has the devastating effect of making social interactions impossible. All students need to do is stare at a screen all day, type questions into a chatbox, or signal for help. Even everyday interactions like socializing after classes, creating groups, illustrative or just hanging out with fellow classmates, are lost. Students can no longer have casual face-to-face conversations with their teachers after classes.

While it might be true that students have video-chat classes and can interact with each other, there is no way to know if the students are actually connected. It's a tool for teachers to host lectures and post assignments. Students lose the opportunity to have a discussion and to learn together.

Slowly, students started adjusting to the realities of the pandemic. If loneliness isn't addressed, it can lead to depression and anxiety in young people.

Poor Academic Performance: According several surveys, nearly half of young students across many demographics learn best when they are surrounded by peers. High engagement levels help them perform well. The lack of regular interaction with peers could lead to poor academic performance even after the pandemic ends. Mental issues such as depression, loneliness and anxiety can all have a major impact on students' academic performance. Students must be aware, diagnosed, and adjusted in a steady manner to return to their normal lives after the pandemic.

The Economic Effects of the Pandemic Upon Millennials

The unluckiest generation in history is the Millennials. They have a large global population. This is because the older generations of millennials hold the majority of the political and decision-making power, while younger millennials are at their peak in education and the labor force.

Why are Millennials so "unlucky?" These reasons are purely economic. The average millennial will likely experience slower economic growth rates than older generations. Gen Z may be a bit more unlucky than millennials, but they have most clearly shown these effects. This generation seems to be worse off than other generations, and it doesn't appear like it will get better any time soon. For instance, only 47.9% U.S. millennials have a home, compared 69% to Gen X, 77.8% to baby boomers, and 78.8% to the silent generation. It's even more worrying because the millennials have a much larger population than any other generation. Economically, the Millennials have a far greater economic advantage than any other generation. This is bad news for mental well-being. Federal Reserve Data indicates that Baby boomers hold over 53% of America's wealth, Gen X holds a little more than 25%, the silent generations controls approximately 17%, and Millennials who form the core of America's working class control only 4.6%.

These statistics are troubling and are correct. However, it's probably more justified that Millennials have been through the most severe economic crisis in their primes. In particular, the 2008 great depression and the COVID-19 pandemic which both had the largest impact on the world's economies in the past century, are the two biggest - guess what? Only Millennials suffered them in their prime work years.

2008 was the year of the recession. The millennials in their twenties were entering the workforce. Since then, this generation has outperformed all negative statistics regarding poor credit due inability to earn wealth, bad debt, unemployment, low-income jobs, mental illness, and inability to pay off their loans. Even though they had higher educational attainments than their parents, they didn't have the same level financial security. It appears that this generation will become poorer in recent times than the older ones.

It doesn't end there. This generation faces more public-health crises as they reach their prime years. It could cause small business failures and make the unemployment crisis worse. While older generations have greater financial security and can bounce back more easily from catastrophes, Millennials are much more vulnerable. They have the lowest jobs, less financial security, fewer assets and homes that can be refinanced. It doesn't end here. This generation also has terrible student-loan debt. The United States has over 500 Billion Dollars in unpaid student loans. They instead work low-skilled, contract jobs and bartending. In times of economic turmoil, those with such low-skill jobs are more at risk of financial troubles. The millennials are therefore unlucky.

Poor financial security and mediocre social standing can have a devastating effect on Millennials mental health. Millennials often suffer from depression due to unpayable credit, bad debt and insufficient wages. To make these meagre wages, they work longer hours. They also experience a lot of stress and burnout. Some of them quit their jobs because they are unhappy with their current job and want to improve their mental health. Although millennials may be less financially able than their older counterparts and have less disposable income, statistics have shown they are more likely that they will pay for therapy sessions than older generations. These people are often called the "therapy Generation."

Millennials are more susceptible to anxiety, depression, stress and burnout than other illnesses.

The American Psychological Association reports that 12 percent of millennials had been diagnosed with an anxiety disorder in 2018. This figure is almost twice that of the baby boomers. According to Blue Cross Blue Shield Association (2018), diagnoses of mental disorders had increased 33 percent over 2013. As you can probably guess, millennials accounted for 47 percent. Some argue that millennials suffer from poor mental well-being because they have been exposed to more horrific events than their elder generations. However the economic consequences that have caused millennials to have poor mental wellbeing cannot be attributed to only a few. It's worse because it leads to poor mental health and poor general health. Life expectancy will continue to decrease worldwide.

Blue Cross Blue Shield Association found that Millennials have experienced a 12% jump in their major depression and a 7% increase to alcohol abuse disorder. There has also been a 5% increase to substance abuse disorder. In 2020, 33% are suffering from behavioral disorders.

This is despite the fact that millennials' mental well-being has always been in question. But, it only got worse in 2020. Why? The short answer: Social isolation.

The pandemic affects all generations, regardless of their age. However the youngest generations are the most affected due to the underlying mental issues society has caused. The state of mental health is on the decline and many are lonely. The reality that many millennials had to live in isolation for quarantine only made matters worse.

A survey done in the United States in 2019 revealed that millennials felt more lonely than any previous generation. Amongst the respondents 30% felt that they were always or often lonely. This is compared to 20% for Gen Xers and 15% for baby boomers. The explanation isn't hard to understand. According to a survey more millennials stated that they didn't know any acquaintances or could refer to them as friends.

These millennials have a lack of meaningful relationships. They have very few people to share ideas with and their interests. Even worse, they have no one with whom to share their emotional struggles. Additionally, millennials are more likely to suffer from social isolation because they are less connected with religious and political communities. Many millennials marry later than their older counterparts, and some don't even get married. This shows that their social support system is already weakening and prolonged periods of social isolation have terribly affected people's mental well-being.

The social disconnect among the younger generation has made the situation worse. It can lead to mental health issues in those living alone, as well as people suffering from anxiety and depression.

Why social isolation has made it worse for the mental health of the younger generation

Millennials are among the youngest generations in the workforce. This implies that they make up the youngest generation to live independently and without their parents. These mental conditions are more severe than for older generations.

The reality is that millennials as well Gen Xers could be at risk of developing mental health problems due to social, environmental and financial trends. These mental illnesses have been exacerbated by social isolation for the following reasons:

* Living Alone. The current pandemic of loneliness amongst millennials has only gotten worse. The majority of working people live alone. One-person apartments are the second most common type in many urban centers. The millennials as well as older Gen Zers live by themselves, which means they have a very predictable life. They move around from home to work, make a few friends there, and then head home. Sometimes they go out with their

girlfriends and boyfriends on weekends. But they prefer to get enough rest most of the day. The good news is that they can meet people daily during times of peak stress. It's possible to laugh with coworkers at work, have productive meetings with their superiors, eat lunch with a friend, or even ride the bus with a few of your acquaintances. This shows that even though they were lonely, young people maintained close contact with friends and maintained meaningful interactions.

However, many people were forced to work from their homes due to the social distancing and pandemic. Only the most essential workers could visit coworkers once a week.

Many are feeling more isolated working from home. The majority of productive people live alone. They spend most of their time on social media, even when they are not resting. Millennials suffered from a shortage in real communication, and many reported mental problems.

Some Millennials, as well as young parents and couples, seem to do better with loneliness than others. They often had children in their late thirties. And they were able to have a wonderful relationship with their spouses. However, only a small proportion of the population is affected by this. Because of their poor social and economic status, most millennials experience slower progress than their older siblings and parents. They reach adult milestones like marriage or childbearing later in life. The loneliness epidemic that millennials are experiencing is worsened by this, especially if they have to stay inside. Remote work was supposed be a way to end the loneliness epidemic. However, working remotely has revealed how poorly millennials have dealt with the pandemic. They have also missed out on socializing in person and have seen how this can have a negative impact on their mental and physical health.

* Longer hours of work: Both loneliness and free-time are interrelated. A 2018 study showed that to be considered a friend, you would need to spend 200 hours together. 200 hours spent together physically, including no texting, no working, just catching up. The millennial generation has worked more hours than the previous generations in order to make ends work. Therefore, they have very little free time. The pandemic was not better. Many people who managed to keep their jobs were too focused on their computers for long hours. They used laptops to conduct meetings and video chats for hours,

making it impossible to have even a small amount of human interaction in the workplace.

People had few friends before and during the pandemic. People are overwhelmed, stressed, and often frustrated. Many people turned to social media to find comfort. However, they were not able to connect with their emotions. While time online is shared, it does not account for quality but only quantity.

While it is great to be able to communicate with colleagues or new friends online, it is not as good as spending time with loved ones. To develop a genuine relationship with people it takes effort, time, as well as physical presence. So the more we don't socialize the better our relationships become. To make matters worse, the more distant and lonely we become, the more serious our mental health becomes. It is important to realize that technology and social networking applications can only keep us connected. They don't create emotional connections. They don't give us emotional connections. That is why we, as social creatures, like to get together face-toface for impromptu parties and hangouts.

\* Unemployment. Despite being educated and having higher levels, Millennials have lower earnings than previous generations. They work less in low-end jobs such as bartending and other jobs that barely allow them to save. Ironically, those low-end jobs will suffer more during the lockdown period when everyone is supposed stay indoors. These jobs are low-end and rely on customer patronage to maximize their sales. Bartenders are not paid if the bars are closed. When people stop eating at restaurants, it is more likely that a restaurant attendant will lose his job. However, many low-end jobs need regular activity to maintain a profit lockdown. In fact, the United States had a record-breaking 10 year unemployment rate.

Unemployment and job loss are not pleasant. People feel insecure and anxious when they have no income. The pandemic caused a surge in job losses over the months that lasted. This has made people feel stressed.

The pandemic has created a lot anxiety and stress due to social distraction and loneliness. People worry about their loved and are afraid of the virus spreading to them. In such difficult times, it seems that people are being forced to accept an unemployment crisis. This is a risky decision. It can also lead to mental health problems.

Previous recessions saw people lose their jobs, which caused economies to collapse and world finances to plummet. People had mental health issues and were able cope with them by having friends and family to talk to. However, the covid epidemic has not only taken away the jobs of those in the working class but also made it impossible for them to find someone to confide in.

People were offered unemployment benefits and stimulus payments by governments all over the world. Some people are forced to take out bad debt in order to survive, despite the lengthy bureaucratic procedures involved in getting these funds. It can get worse when people make mistakes with their information for the stimulus checks. They may not receive the correct information for months. A combination of poor financial situation and social isolation often destroys self-confidence, as well as a person's sense of identity. These mental health effects can be long-lasting after the pandemic.

## The Pandemic Pandemic: Social Media's Effects on Social Isolation and Loneliness

Many young people have found social media to be a refuge. Social media is especially popular with people below 40 years of old. This is not surprising, since this group tends to be the most disconnected and isolated. When we are always connected to others via social media, it is not surprising that many of us feel disconnected. It is ironic that, despite having the means and ability to stay connected with others, millennials/Gen Zers feel more alone than older generations.

Social media and the Internet offer faster communication and a way for people to stay connected anywhere, anytime. The Internet is a way to communicate faster, but it's not a replacement for genuine bonding and connection. Many teenagers use the Internet incorrectly. These social networks are great for staying in touch with friends and reaching people without physically visiting them. Spending hours each day trying to connect with people via social media will only make you feel worse.

It's common for social anxious people to use social media apps to get temporary relief. This feeling of happiness, however, can become toxic. Because the connection was never established, this feeling of connection fades. It is only a social construct which promotes temporary happiness.

In addition, social media creates false expectations of happiness. By looking at the updates of friends on social media, one might think that this person is happy and fulfilled. However, subconsciously, they see other people's lives and assume that their life is more interesting than theirs.

Many social media users desire a perfect life, with no problems. The ideal life is one where everything is planned and it is possible to live happily ever afterwards. Many social media users are inclined to believe that everyone they see online has a perfect life. Then self-esteem problems begin to surface. People often have social media icons they admire and want to be like. In turn, they start to compare themselves to other social media users, trying to get likes and comments. They also monitor the number of people sending them "happy birthday wishes". If it is less than their preferred benchmark they assume they are not loved enough.

It's a shame to discover that, despite all the attempts at faux happiness on social networks, loneliness and despair are still serious issues in this day.

According to data, both millennials as well as older Gen Zers use social media more than other generations. An average millennial spends three hours per day on social networks. The highest number of users visits the platforms more often than 50 times per week. Unfortunately, this generation is stuck in routines. They just want to go to work or school, then get home to tweet. The problem is that some addicts use their free time to chat with virtual friends online and find friendships more difficult offline.

I was helping a younger friend out of a complete mental and social block. She was a young woman of 27 who had been shy, dare i say, since birth. Susan will be my surname for confidentiality and trust.

Susan thought social media was a way to engage with the world. Susan felt it was a way of reaching out to people she did not feel comfortable with. Susan was shy, so it was hard to make friends. My guesses are as valid as mine. Susan was obsessed by social media and was constantly distracted. She averaged 8 hours a days on social media with active accounts for all the platforms. For her, it was a way to be connected and happy. At first, she did not spend more than 2 hours each day on social networking. But she claims that the moment she dropped her smartphone, she felt empty. She then went back to social networks like a drug addict. At first she thought she was fighting loneliness by using social media. Susan felt that her inability of connecting with people face-to-face could be replaced by staying connected online. She felt even more depressed and rejected the more she spent her time on the timeline. She felt excluded when her "friends" never reached out. She was the one constantly trying to keep up. She saw posts about events and even photos from them, but she never got invited.

Susan expected increased social media usage to give her the feeling of having a community of friends. However, she found that it was a distraction from her loneliness, and made her feel even more vulnerable to rejection.

Susan craved approval and validation, just as many social media junkies who are obsessed with getting a thousand likes for their posts. I told her she could only heal from the horrible feeling she experienced and her dependency on others to validate her feelings. I advised her to "know who you are and what you're worth." Don't wait for anyone to tell you how gorgeous you are on Facebook. To build your self worth and your ego, you must first reduce your social media usage.

Susan felt like everything was going to fall apart. She asked her how she could survive if she wasn't spending long hours online. She explained that she could not maintain her sanity if she was not online. So I sat with her and explained to her how social media addiction has affected her. She showed signs of rejection and depression, loneliness and low self-esteem.

It was a difficult task as she spent 8+ hours each day on social networks. I told her to cut down to an hour daily. I advised her that she use apps that track screen time and that she can revoke access to such apps if it exceeds an hour.

It felt as if I was asking her for the whole world. She found it extremely difficult to adjust. I was able to see it coming. She will need to fill the seven hour gap with her own content. I suggested that she get more connected with the real-world to help her make up for her social media withdrawal.

With a little help, she got back on track and joined a support team. Susan was determined to make friends and not be alone. There she discovered that socializing doesn't mean hanging out in bars and going to parties. However, she was able to find people who could identify and connect with her, which gave her the opportunity to feel a sense of genuine connection and intimacy offline. Her colleagues had low self-esteem and social isolation, so the support group helped them identify recreational activities that they could enjoy together. Susan became interested in badminton and joined a music group. As time went by, her addiction began to subdue and she was happy.

Even though she used social media, it was to check up on friends and family she had through her physical connections, as well as her musical partners and her colleagues. She found that social media allowed her to share with others what was happening in the day. In just a few months, she became confident in her social media skills. She even helped other members of the support group identify their Weaknesses.

Sharing this story is meant to help you understand that social networking is a tool for strengthening our offline connections and not a replacement for real human connection and interaction.

In times of social isolation where it's impossible to visit clubs and you can not stay with your teammates for casual sporting events or go to work, you will find that social media appeals to you and becomes even more appealing. What should you do?

During extended periods of isolation and quarantine many people increased their dependency on social media as a source of entertainment and information. Social media is meant to be fun, and it can also help you relax after long periods of stress. It is alarming that this tool is often misused, especially among millennials. It is very interesting that people under 40, usually millennials, have a higher percentage of social media users than the rest. Surveys that examine gender, race, or other sensitive factors show that increased use of social media is a recipe to loneliness.

As you likely know, loneliness is a serious problem that has plagued people since long before COVID-19. Today, isolation is worsened by the increasing dependence on social media.

Good interpersonal relationships must be mutually beneficial. During the lockdown people were asked not to leave their homes and maintained social distance. This led to many people trying to make attachments to people that they didn't know. It's not human nature to connect with strangers at first contact.

Man's attachment to family and close knit circles has existed since primitive times.

However, Millennials do not have a true community and circle to which to reach out. They are less likely to be involved in political and religious groups, as well as community gatherings. These relationships were a way for older people to keep in touch with their loved ones, especially those who are involved in politics or religion. Millennials feel isolated during this time. Their social platforms are not used to meet up with friends or colleagues. But, like Susan, they seek to establish new connections and make new connections with others.

Most people don't make connections through social media. Most people create a utopia on social media - a life that is perfect for them to face the fear of the pandemic. They resort to social media to replace their need for connection. Unfortunately, they are unable to stop using it and the data that they have wasted is not sufficient to fill the void.

## Chapter 4: The Relationship Between Mental Health, Happiness, Needs And Needs

Abraham Maslow was an American psychologist who developed a theory of decision-making for humans in 1943. This theory was linked to Maslow's psychological needs and presented a hierarchy. Maslow claims that five kinds of human needs drive or motivate actions. Abraham Maslow's theory posited that every person has five basic human needs. These need include safety, love, belonging and self-actualization.

Maslow's law holds that each category plays a significant role in human decision-making and that they are ranked according to their importance. To help fuel healthy human behavior, basic human necessities like water, shelter, warmth and sleep are important.

Think about it for a moment. The likelihood is that you will make bad decisions because you have to stop eating due to a pandemic. This has caused people to needlessly dip into their long-term financial plans. They are now focusing on what they can do right now.

The Maslow Pyramid

Maslow says that human behavior is influenced by these needs. Unfortunately, the pandemic halted normal life and caused reduced income or none, disruptions to sleeping patterns, anxiety over infection, and worries about the safety of their health. Many people are affected physiologically by these fears, and their behavior has changed in order to deal with them.

This means that when someone is in extreme need of food and shelter, security, and safety across all ramifications, it becomes more likely that their behavior will change. They will feel a void and then attempt to fill it with various coping mechanisms, both healthy and unhealthy.

Higher up Maslow's pyramid are higher human needs, such as self-esteem, self-actualization and potential realization. These needs are affected directly by financial stability, income, family, education success, and work. Human needs are not satisfied. It is a common misconception that human wants can be insatiable. Our human nature is to always be in need of some thing. These needs are often not caused by lack, but from an innate desire for growth.

Abraham Maslow (the Philosopher) pointed out that the pyramid was not rigid and does not necessarily follow the progression. Although it does in most cases, it is not. There are many different people with different outlooks and desires. We all have different needs. For example, people may have different needs depending on their financial status. One person may be focused only on safety, security, and love while the other person may be more focused on self-actualization, creativity, esteem and creativity.

No matter the type, everyone is affected by the pandemic. It is now obvious that their physical, financial, as well as emotional needs are urgent. Many suffer from mental illness because they feel too weak and ineffective to deal with these needs. Let's discuss each level of mental health need and how it has been affected by the pandemic.

Security and Safety Needs. The human need for safety and security is essential. People crave financial security. People desire financial security.

People are looking for work, starting a company, learning soft skills, or trading to provide specific services in order to achieve financial stability. Financial security is essential for everyone. A lack of income can cause depression. Research has shown that low income can lead to unhappiness and depression. Insecure feelings can set in when there is no steady income. People may feel financially handicapped or disabled without a stable source of income. Financial insecurity was high after the COVID-19 Pandemic. Many businesses laid off workers, some reduced payment, and many businesses couldn't operate because of this social isolation. Many artisans were also unable to make a living due to the ban on people visiting others. Slowly, but surely people had to dip into their savings to make sure they could eat properly and have access health care. Many people had health insurance coverage before the pandemic. But, once they lost their income due to the financial crisis, depression and widespread unhappiness were common.

It was so bad that many people couldn't afford their rent anymore. They had no choice but to leave their home and find shelter in unfamiliar areas.

These examples demonstrate the effect of the pandemic as well as social isolation on our security, safety and needs. People are feeling more anxious and needy than ever, with their mental wellbeing suffering.

Social Needs - As we said, humans are social animals. We all want love, connection, acceptance and a sense that we belong. Happiness is directly related to how our social needs and well-being are met. You already know that happiness is key to good mental health. People make friends, form relationships with others, share their love with extended families members, and even join religious and social groups in order to fit in with the smaller communities. These communities are usually worth the effort because they offer love, friendship, engaging conversations, and hangouts. These communities often provide happiness for many.

I once had the pleasure of consulting with a woman that was a Christian and a Christian follower. During many of our conversations, I learned that she had reservations about the Christian faith. She believes some Christian beliefs are too extreme or unrealistic for today's society. I asked her if she felt these things would make her less inclined to participate in church programs. But, she said no. She enjoyed the social aspect of church and made many new friends. She was also a member of sub-groups within the church. These groups provided a great way to meet social needs. According to her, these groups made her feel alive and happy. Despite her disagreements with certain religious beliefs, she would prefer to stay in the community since it satisfied her social needs.

It is not news that the social isolation caused by the pandemic as well as the stay-at home guidelines has discouraged many people from maintaining their social connections. It's worse for millennials. They make up the bulk and majority of the working age population.

Social isolation is now mandatory. Because of this, you are restricted from going to clubs, religious gatherings, or even participating in recreational activities. Even worse, if you don't live with your partner, it means you don't get the chance to see them. The social gap keeps growing. Many people become socially isolated, unhappy, and depressed because of this. These people attempt to deal with these drastic changes and their mental health suffers.

Abraham Maslow describes Esteem as the need to show appreciation for loved ones, colleagues, friends, and families. In order to have positive self-esteem, and self-worth, we need to be valued and respected by others. People are more likely to be recognized and acknowledged for certain achievements. These achievements could include accomplishments in the community, at school, or other activities that bring happiness to their family. Recognition and praises from others are often a way for people to satisfy their self-esteem. People who don't have the ability to appreciate and respect others start to feel inferior and develop low self-esteem.

This may be partially due to the lack or financial security associated with the pandemic. Many people, particularly the working-class, are breadwinners to family members, siblings and close friends. But when they don't earn as much, or lose their income completely, they start to lose self-esteem. They are no more able to provide for their loved ones, they cannot satisfy them and this can affect their mental health.

Other people, including professional athletes, feel their life has been stopped.

They need to go home. It is difficult to set new records or smash old ones and achieve new accomplishments. As a result, their timelines for reaching milestones have all been destroyed. They feel like they have been left in the same place and are unable to make any further progress. It can be difficult to get the appreciation of co-workers for solving problems when you are not physically present. Simply put, the motivation to do even more vanishes.

Social and esteem problems are the most severe effects of the pandemic. These issues directly relate to the psychology of people, making them more harmful to mental well-being.

Self-Actualization Needs. Self-actualization can be described as the pinnacle of human need, but not everyone will get there. Self-actualization happens when people feel they have achieved all they can but still feel they need to fulfill their full potential.

People who are financially stable, successful, and seem to have everything under control are the ones who tend to have self-actualization needs. Even though they have achieved great success, many people still feel like they aren't fully exploring their abilities and talents. They feel they can't reach their full potential and must work harder to achieve it. People experience a temporary sense of satisfaction that is short-lived.

However, it is very unfortunate that the pandemic left many people feeling depressed. They cannot continue to work to achieve this feeling of satisfaction and can only sit at home following the rules and remaining unproductive.

Even for seemingly successful people, this feeling can also lead to unhappiness and depression. They want to do more, be better and achieve greater things, but they feel stuck because of their isolation from others.

Happiness, Mental Health

Happiness is the state of being happy. It's a feeling of joy or well-being when people achieve their desires and needs. Happiness can be found when the innate human desires are fulfilled. People therefore live their lives seeking to fulfill their natural desires, become rich, have better relationships, travel the world, be happier, and to make their lives easier. It's not news that the COVID-19 virus pandemic has led to decreased happiness. People can't fulfill all their wants, needs, or desires and are left unhappy, stressed, and depressed.

It is not uncommon for people to fail to recognize that mental stress can cause as much stress as physical stress. According to medical research it has been found that mental illness occurs in the same brain region as physical illnesses. Even worse, it can cause permanent disability. It is difficult to see with the eyes and can cause even more damage than physical pain. It happens that you are able to see the mark immediately after you have struck your feet against the wall. Even if there is physical discomfort, the cause can be determined and treated. You may need to test your internal organs in order to make a diagnosis. Physical illnesses can also be diagnosed with MRI Scans (CTI Scans), X-rays, or other equipment. To identify mental illness, you will need to do a deeper analysis and self-evaluation. Mental illnesses and physical illnesses can be treated in different ways.

A majority of people with mental illnesses get immediate treatment, but a significant number of people with mental illnesses don't receive any treatment at all.

People feel sad, unhappy, and depressed from a lack of fulfillment in their lives. This reality became more stark during the pandemic. As people were forced into finding ways to satisfy their neediness, many became unhappy. It is common for people to feel that some needs are more important than others. A person may not feel the same way as you.

Fortunately, all of us were able to adapt to different situations during the pandemic. Our brains are wired for survival and growth in even the most severe conditions. This kind of approach to life makes us more hungry for our emotions. As we begin to realize that positive experiences that give us joy are very common, we find that our need for more happiness becomes more normal. Many people didn't feel the emotional fulfillment they expected after the pandemic. It was because their initial happiness level has been raised.

Many people feel that the pandemic left them feeling empty. They want to be more successful, wealthy, influential, popular, and so forth. Mental health cannot be switched off. You can switch it off and back on whenever you like. However, mental illness accumulates over time. And your return to mental wellbeing will only happen if you make conscious efforts. You cannot chase happiness and all the things society says it is. Seek out happiness that is not based on immediate, drastic changes. Instead, focus on finding true happiness by fulfilling your natural needs.

Tips for Remaining Happy Even During the Social Isolation Period

Maintain Positivity. One survival strategy that men have used for thousands of years is to identify, observe, and recall negative things or things that do not make sense. This method has been used since primitive men, when they needed to be able to remember dangerous patterns in order stay safe in a world full of physical stress. This trait is unfortunately inherited from evolution. Our brains can detect all the wrong things before they are even noticed. This trait is often a cause of mental stress, and even unhappiness. It is true that genetics cannot be changed and it is impossible to alter the natural flight and fight mechanisms. However, positive thinking can be taught to our brains.

Maintaining positivity can't be a substitute to confronting reality. You can identify situations where things aren't going well and take steps to improve them. But, positive thinking doesn't necessarily mean negative thoughts should be avoided.

Express your gratitude: Several studies have demonstrated that genuine happiness is linked to gratitude. It is possible to be grateful for the little things that you have, which will help you feel positive and relieve depression. A grateful attitude will make you more efficient in your spending. You can express gratitude or appreciation in many different ways.

* Appreciate Others. When someone is willing to go the extra mile to help you,

they should be thanked with a heartfelt thank you. This makes both you and them feel great and gives you an inner lift. Gratitude will always make someone feel better about you. It can also bring you inner joy. All of us are interconnected and whatever good thing you get will make someone else happy.

* Start journaling: Now you may be laughing at the idea of keeping a journal, even though you're not meeting all your needs. But it's always helpful to take a moment to notice and record the good things that happen every day. It directs your subconscious mind to think only about positive events. When you do this, the feeling of happiness quickly overwhelms the feeling of depression. You feel happier and more connected to others. You might wonder if you have much to be grateful. I still believe that you should count your blessings.

Regardless of how small they may seem, reflect on them and think about how they can help you through your day. You'll be amazed at how valuable they are and why you should appreciate them.

* Be grateful for long-term kindnesses: We have had many people help us with our needs. There are certain circumstances that may have prevented you being able to properly thank the person. It is possible to write a letter to express your gratitude to the person. You could then, if possible, physically walk up to the person to read the contents and let them know that you appreciate their efforts. Reciprocal appreciation could be possible if you show gratitude.

* Make Lemonades Out of Lemons. It is important to find the positives that you can draw from a negative experience and

to be grateful. Even the most terrible circumstances can teach you valuable lessons. These past events should be viewed objectively and the lessons learned. When you are able to distinguish the good from the ugly, you will be happier and more appreciative.

Treat Relationships Like Gold: Investing our time and money in our relationships is one the most profitable investments we can make. Healthy relationships can lead to happiness. Humans are social creatures. Therefore, it is easier to feel happy when you have good social support. Your happiness will increase if your relationships are strong with your loved ones and you have a good social life. This is a worthwhile endeavor that you won't regret. When you put in the effort to build positive relationships, you will quickly feel happier and be able to help others. Here are some things to consider when building relationships.

* Stay Connected. While we are all busy working to make money and build careers, we must not forget to keep in touch with our loved ones. This is one of few things that gives life meaning. Being surrounded with people you love is a wonderful way to relax and eliminate stress. If you are willing to put in the effort, it is possible to stay in touch today with people. You can write to friends, call and visit them in person. Your physical presence can make you a happier person by building a stronger and more friendly relationship.

Spend less time on the phone, texting, or in front the TV and more quality time with the people that matter to you. You can share the things you are worried about and listen to what they have to say. Get out with friends and have fun. Keep in mind that it's the quality of your time that is important and not how many you spend.

* Give compliments to other people: Complimenting others is an important part of building relationships. If you look at your friends, you'll notice admirable qualities. Give compliments, laud them for their efforts, and appreciate their friendship. You will find that such people are happier and more inclined to become a good friend. You will appreciate your relationship and it will grow in value. This will lead to greater happiness.

* Hang out with happy people. Emotions can spread like a virus. It's a good idea to spend time with people who are always happy, understand their reasons for happiness, and show genuine interest in them. React positively to their happiness

and be happy for the others around you. You shouldn't be sad or feel threatened by happy people. Instead, you should show genuine enthusiasm and love for those close to you who experience good fortune. Do not be jealous, envious, or compete with others for the sake of feeling better. Instead, try to share in their happiness, pay attention, ask queries, and be excited. If you truly invest in the happiness others have, you will also discover good news.

Keep Your Eyes on the Present. It's okay for you to live in today and still enjoy your life. But if you start to think about the future too often, you can end up worrying, having high expectations and fear of failure. These kinds of thoughts could lead to depression. Your life will lose its meaning if you think too much about the future. It is better just to live in the now. This will increase your chances of noticing the good things you have right now and not letting them slip by you because you worry too much about the future. So, how do you live in this moment and appreciate the wonderful things in life?

* Try Meditation: Mindful meditation is a wonderful technique for meditating and allowing yourself to enjoy the moment. Experts recommend meditation as an exercise that is good for the brain. Meditation, when practiced regularly, tends to eliminate negative, depressing, sad, and anxious brain activities. While increasing brain activities that relate to happiness and joy, peace and satisfaction, it can be a healthy exercise for the brain.

* Be a part of Daily Routines. Choose something you love and do it every morning. You can do it all, whether you

are walking with your dog or shopping at the grocery store, or participating in some other activity. Make sure you engage in it every single day. It doesn't make a difference what you do. Do it daily if it makes you smile. You will find happiness and a better way to live your life.

* Savour Pleasant Memories: Reminiscing about pleasant memories and happy experiences from the past can help you build more positive emotions for today. You shouldn't rush to forget the pleasant moments. Keep a log, record videos and photos, and enjoy these moments. It will make you happy. It is possible to take a break and appreciate the memories you have.

Engage In Purposeful Volunteering. As I stated earlier, the only way to feel fulfilled is when you can see that your actions have a positive impact on the world. This is why charitable organizations are so popular. These groups help people make a positive difference in the world and give back. It creates a sense that people are responsible and brings joy. It is the reason why everyone, from the lowest income earners to billionaires, are willing to do whatever they can to help the poor. It is fulfilling to help others. Your actions will be a big part of their relief. It's okay to feel like you are making an impact in the world. How can you make it happen?

* Volunteering - When you volunteer, you are actively helping others. Such activities could include counseling/mentoring, walking kids home from school, fostering animal shelters, etc. Even if your donation is only a few hundred dollars it will make a

difference in the life of someone else. Doing this will allow you to take the first step towards self-actualization, and ultimately lead you to true happiness.

Random Acts of Kindness: Don't feel pressure to find a charity before making a difference in the world. Helping a stranger with their extra luggage is a great way to make them happy. If you have the time, reduce their workload and go out of your ways to do a favor. Random acts of kindness that don't require any preparation are often appreciated and cherished. It brings joy to you, it increases your self-esteem and makes you feel happy.

* Never forget that you can't do it all: You must always remember that God cannot be played. Your strengths should guide your activities. Building around your loyalty, for example, is a great way

to build. If you're funny, build around that. Do not try to help people by trying to make it easier for them. This will cause you to fail and leave you feeling unhappy, unfulfilled and depressed.

Be Conscious About Your Health: Exercise and sleep are important factors that you can control. Good sleep and exercise are essential for your mental and physical health. Happyness can also be linked to exercise and good sleep habits. Healthy living requires regular, healthy exercise as well as adequate sleep.

Happiness is a key ingredient in physical health

Medicine has known for a long time that happiness and mental health are closely related. It is how positive emotions can lead to happiness. Happiness also helps us avoid anxiety and depression. Many links have not been made between happiness and our physical health. Many studies have demonstrated that emotions, positive and negative, can have an impact on our lives in ways we don't even realize.

It is also interrelated because poor mental and physical health can lead to mental problems. Indirectly, poor mental outlook could lead to mental problems.

John Hopkins University School of Medicine surveyed 1,500 people and found that happiness, positive emotions, optimism, fulfillment, and happiness contributed to a 30% decline in heart disease. The study was followed by 1,500 sibling with a history of high-risk heart disease. This study showed that the 50% of people most at risk of developing these heart diseases were those who displayed positive emotions. Medical research has also shown that happiness reduces hypertension risk by stabilizing the heart rate and blood pressure.

Research has shown that happiness and immune system strength are linked. Studies have shown that people who feel positive emotions are more likely to recover from illness. Medical researchers discovered that people who have positive emotions and eliminated fear had stronger immune systems. This indicates that people who are happy and optimistic about their lives face a significantly lower chance of getting sick than people who are anxious or angry.

Last but not least, happiness and positive emotions have strong links with long life. Many studies have shown that those with positive emotions outlive their peers more than those who are unhappy and dissatisfied.

You could go on, but the evidence is overwhelming that happy people tend to be healthier mentally and physically. We know that people who are physically active and socially connected are often healthier. So happiness, even if it isn't isolated, contributes to good emotional well being. It also helps to build better mental and social relationships. It can help people overcome depression and anxiousness.

People who are content and happy with their lives are less likely use harmful coping mechanisms, such as emotional eating or substance abuse. This can pose a serious threat to their physical health.

Our choices eventually make us victims. Even though we cannot control our environment, genetic and other factors, everything that can affect our mental and physical health is within our reach.

You cannot separate your lifestyle choices from your health. That is why it is crucial to make conscious choices to live happy and fulfilled lives. Fulfilling our self-actualization goals and self-esteem is as important a goal as taking care our psychological, and physiological needs.

In fact, laughter is the best medicine. Without a doubt, needs and happiness are interconnected. Mental health is dependent on maintaining a high level if happiness.

Coping mechanisms for social isolation

Before the pandemic, everyone had experienced stress. People may also be under pressure at work because of their performance, their relationships or other issues. Whatever the case may have been, stress is a normal part of life.

When people feel stressed, lonely, depressed, or anxious, they seek out ways to relieve themselves. These outlets could be beneficial or detrimental to the mind and body. Unfortunately, many people don't realize how harmful their practices can be. This is why people seek out quick solutions when they desperately need them.

There are healthy coping methods to deal with loneliness and stress during the pandemic. Some people found a new hobby and started knitting. Others were more active to keep fit. People can also engage in self-meditation to manage stress. Some people find solace in destructive behaviors like self-medication or alcohol. Others eat excessively to alleviate stress related financial, psychological, and physical issues. It is concerning that these unhealthy coping methods will not be addressed once the lockdown has ended.

## Chapter 5: Self-Medication is a Coping Tool

As the pandemic progressed, people were placed in lockdown situations for longer periods. This led to feelings like loneliness, anxiety and boredom. These feelings seem to have remained despite the difficult experiences of millennials. This is why the COVID-19 Pandemic came as a natural trigger. People look for ways to deal and feel "alive" and self-medication can be a great option. To deal with the mental rigors caused by the pandemic, many people turn to drugs and alcohol for comfort.

It is likely that a couple of glasses of wine or a bottle beer will not cause any problems, especially if there has been no underlying medical condition. Self-medication, especially when it comes to substance use, can often be used as a quick fix for anxiety. However, an excessive intake can cause mental problems that are worse. This makes it less effective and causes people to feel worse. The effects also last for a longer time, even after the pandemic.

This "habit" (or coping mechanism) was quite common during pandemic. Numerous researchers reported a notable increase in substance use in young adults and teens to improve their mood. Others who don't use alcohol or substance abuse excessively in order to lift their moods and avoid boredom. From smoking a few joints to drinking a few alcoholic beverages for relaxation, substance abuse can be started by using a few joints. It gets worse as people use antidepressants to induce sleeping and ADHD medication to stay awake during the day, or opioids in order to cope with the pandemic.

People know that they have mental problems, but avoid the healthy ways to deal with them. Self-medication is temporary and may provide some comfort in the short term. However, it can actually lead to more mental health problems.

Frequent, indiscriminate self-medication can lead you to addiction, unhappiness, or even compromise your general well-being. As you become more dependent on the substance, you could end up severing meaningful relationships and even excluding yourself from others.

Self-medication is available in a variety of forms

* Alcohol: The availability of alcohol makes it easy to abuse. Many reports have confirmed that alcohol intake has been increasing exponentially during the pandemic. Many people use them to

self-medicate stress, depression, anxiety. This is as bad as shooting oneself in a foot. Alcohol, beer, wine, liquor and all other forms of alcohol are depressants.

\* Drugs. Many people resort to using prescription drugs like opioids and ADHD medications to combat stress and sleeplessness. These drugs can help you concentrate, especially when you work remotely. These drugs can be easily abused and are readily available.

Some people take indiscriminate use of recreational drugs such as cannabis and marijuana. Some people use stronger drugs such as heroin, cocaine and other stimulants. Amphetamines are sometimes used by people to deal with PTSD and other unpleasant emotions. Unfortunately, drug abuse and addiction can result from increased prescription or recreational use. Expert efforts are required to get rid of this problem long after the pandemic.

Excessive eating: This is an effective way to combat stress, anxiety and unpleasant feelings. When they are trapped with food in their homes, it's not unusual for them to turn to food for comfort when they have mental health problems. However, emotional eating can become a routine and lead to unhealthy eating habits that can lead to insecurity and mood swings.

Cigarettes - Nicotine, which is a substance in cigarettes, and other tobacco products, triggers a neurotransmitter known as "dopamine" that provides temporary joy and helps to overcome anxiety and stress. The downside to tobacco and nicotine is that they can be addictive and dependent. These people also tend to experience worse ADHD symptoms and may find it more difficult to quit smoking.

## Substance abuse during and after pandemics: the dangers

A pattern of indeliberate use or abuse of drugs, substances, alcohol, or other substances can make it worse. These temporary solutions only serve to exacerbate existing problems. The depressive feelings come back once the numbing effects stop. The effects of self-medicating or substance abuse on sleep, immunity and energy levels as well as susceptibility for diseases and other illnesses can be significant. Slowly and steadily, the abuser falls into a deep depression due to repeated poor-substance mood worsening that leads to increased substance abuse. It is quite ironic, that it takes more self-medication to find some relief. Addiction becomes a problem. You might need three beers to feel numb. Once you get over your initial anxiety, your tolerance to beer will grow. For the same amount of relief, you might need five beers. Your tolerance will increase, your addiction will worsen, and you'll have more problems due to your new found habit. It's a vicious cycle that can only be broken with healthier coping mechanisms.

Since the pandemic, many people have been caught up in this vicious circle and are still trying to escape. However, the problem got worse and stress didn't seem able to go away. They feel more alone than they did during pandemic.

Many suffer from anxiety and addiction. Many people find themselves in deeper financial trouble due to over-spending on drugs.

These bad habits eventually lead to more mental health issues. There are some people who have had mental health problems in the past. These addictions might lead to additional mental health issues. Medical research has shown that increased Opioid and alcohol intake can cause depression.

## Chapter 6: The Pandemic And Its Dangers For Social Relations

Humans are social creatures, with many beliefs, prejudices, or values. Culture and history is as old as tribes.

Fear, prejudices, or discrimination have always been part of human history. Many people attribute the spread to others' actions. Others believe that the pandemic has been a result of religious punishment. Still others believe that it is simply a power struggle between the big guns.

This backlash often targets minority and disadvantaged groups. A simple example is how Native Americans refer the COVID-19 Virus to as the "Chinese Virus", in an attempt to give a prejudicial explanation that fits their beliefs. But, this spread of discrimination and conspiracy theory only leads to irredeemable social frictions which cause many other reactions, especially mental health problems.

COVID-19 caused a panic among people because it spreads faster than any other viruses and bacteria breakouts such as Ebola, MERS, SARS and Ebola.

Discrimination, stigmatization and exclusion of patients who have recovered from the flu became a problem, while conspiracy theories about the virus and vaccine became a legitimate concern for mental health. Ostracization and discrimination are just as old as racial diversity. We witness this every day in our neighbourhoods, schools and workplaces. Experts have also shown that they have adverse effects on relationships and psychological well being (especially in the most disadvantaged communities).

These can manifest in many ways: verbal and contextual discrimination; name-calling, exclusion hostility, cyberbullying; obscene gestures; scapegoating, harassment or even physical violence. This is not proper and causes victims to feel isolated and rejected.

These socially dangerous acts are usually rooted in prejudice. They are often based on long-standing experience, mostly historical. Prejudice is a dangerous agenda that leads to discrimination and mental illness.

* Stigmatization. It is an ancient social construct that people have displayed, even among the most educated. It is easy to see how stigmatization and social rejection have led to the emergence of mental illnesses in HIV/AIDS survivors. The first thing that stigmatization does to the body is to create fear. People don't

want people to find out their status. They feel unsafe. They fear that a slight error could cause them to be abandoned by loved ones or family. These thoughts can stress the mind. After treatment and quarantine, those who became infected by the virus experienced several Stigmatization mechanisms from family and friends. People become silent, stop communicating and go AWOL. You don't hear anything from them anymore. People are treated as potential murderers or tainted. They receive harsh words, as well as negative reactions.

Despite their obvious recovery and treatment some people refuse their association with them, which negatively affects their mental health. In fact, some countries have established support groups to help COVID survivors.

This stigmatization even extended to healthcare workers. Some people believe they might be virus carriers, and certain communities like Asian-Americans have been the victims of violence and discrimination. Some people have lost work after testing positive. This combined with other factors made the mental health threats during the pandemic worse than the pandemic itself.

Stigma is detrimental to both mental and physical well-being. In fact, it has been shown that chronic stress can lead to cardiovascular and heart disease.

Stigma can affect even people who don't have a social prejudice. A light cough in the shopping center could make people move 10m away. Others could leave the whole room, as they are afraid of getting infected. These factors all combine to destroy people's mental health.

* Conspiracy Theories. To believe in something we need to find explanations that are beyond their comprehension. They don't care about how plausible the beliefs are. They don't care about the plausibility of the beliefs as long it provides answers to questions that have baffled their minds. These beliefs can be religiously based, political, or even with some scientific background. The main purpose of these beliefs is to fill the void caused by confusion and uncertainty. Humans are driven by a strong desire to make everything understandable. When people don't have the answers, they create them, spreading these falsehoods across the globe.

These conspiracy theory creators attempt to control their mentality in the midst of chaos. They come up with answers to seemingly unrelated questions just to feel sane. This is why it's common to consider this a coping mechanism. This coping mechanism is driven by misinformation and distortion, which spread fear, uncertainty and tension among ordinary people. This can lead to deeper mental disorders. These theories are generally disproven with solid evidence. However, those desperate for explanations stick to theories that are easily shared on social media.

Another reason these conspiracy Theories fly so easily is because people are looking for scapegoats. They will point fingers at a group of people who are responsible for the economic destruction that the pandemic has caused. Even though there was no proof of the disease being genetically engineered, many believed that it was a tool to promote political war. This explains the stigmatization of Asian-Americans and the ostracization they have experienced during this period. Many people blame them and some suffer severe mental health issues. They also refuse to make contact with many people due to paranoia. This discrimination and stigmatization have led to some of them losing their jobs.

It is easy for conspiracy writers to point fingers at the wealthy and powerful in order to make some sense of the virus. Bill Gates is often referred to as the "devil's agent", who is trying in vain to implant tracking technology disguised as vaccines to control people and gain access to their data. Because they don't want microchips in their bodies, some who have taken the vaccine are anxious. Recently, I came across a video where a woman claimed to possess magnetic arms. This was done to prove that Bill Gates and Fauci were the original creators of this virus.

Many other bizarre conspiracy theories were circulated. These included encouraging people not use masks, encouraging them not to get vaccinated and demonizing some people. This is the crazy thing about all of this: millions of people believe these ridiculous theories. I once found the Twitter comment section for a Bill Gates posting, where several hate speech and verbal abuses were directed at him as the original cause of the pandemic.

Contrary to people's expectations and beliefs, studies have shown that those who believe and follow conspiracy theories are more likely suffer from mental distress. These conspiracy theories were a major hindrance to the control of this virus, and they led to widespread mental health decline. Many studies have also shown that anxiety levels were elevated when people believe in these conspiracy theories.

These beliefs can also create a negative bias in people and lead them to believe that others are evil, satanic, or hostile. This paranoia can lead them to feel that they are victims of other people. Unfortunately, these mental disorders can persist long after the pandemic.

It gets worse. It gets worse. Many people start to look for conspiracy theories on the Internet. They find a community of like-minded believers that claim to have discovered all the secrets in the world. They start to become paranoid and begin to lose touch with their families. These people look for information that doesn't relate to each other and combine them to appeal to more people. They believe it to be true and spread dangerously falsehoods.

Another study has shown that conspiracy theories make it worse for people who have psychological imbalances. Many people have psychological issues that cannot be met. Therefore, in order to keep a healthy balance they need to gain a better understanding of the world. These conspiracy theories provide them with some kind of explanation and a greater sense of satisfaction.

Studies in the past have shown that conspiracy theories can be associated with anxiety and social isolation. The COVID-19 panic caused a new wave in research that suggests there may be a link between anxiety, depression, uncertainty, and conspiracy theories.

Multiple studies and reports have revealed that many people who believe this twisted information are anxious about finding the next doom. They become less sane and have trouble relating to their friends, family, and co-workers over these bizarre beliefs. They become isolated and feel more alone. Their mental health declined, even though they were in a good place before they began to get involved in the absurd beliefs. How can you have healthy relationships with someone who believes in evil, flesh-eating and satanic pedophiles that want to be the savior? This made little sense and people who have been indoctrinated into such cults often become disillusioned. For such people, loneliness, anxiety, bipolar disorders and many other mental disorders are just the beginning. Long after the pandemic, these beliefs continue to be held, connecting dots that don't exist in order to prove the existence of a conspiracy or enemy.

These people often experience deep trauma. Sometimes their mental health deteriorates to the point where they have severe mental health conditions, such as schizophrenia or post-traumatic stress syndrome (PTSD), bipolar disorder, and hundreds more.

Your New Journey

Simply by purchasing this book, you are already a big step closer to your goal of mental wellness. Finding the will and drive to exercise is one of the greatest hurdles that people face. You already have the desire to make progress and take action, as you can see by reading these pages. You already have something to be proud.

It is not difficult to see that life is full of negative experiences. Many times, these can inflict some pain on us. While it is inevitable, we do not need to be controlled by this fact. We often allow ourselves too easily to be controlled or influenced by negative aspects of our lives. It can lead to negative beliefs and habits in our mind. Our minds can be filled with negative thoughts, such as the fear that we will not be able do certain things or that our goal is impossible. These thoughts can lead to us staying stuck.

The media is a huge influencer on negative feelings and thoughts. This includes both national and online media. We see the bad things going around the world and it can take all of our optimism away. It is rare that national news reports on positive developments around the world. This means we are just being fed negativity. Social media encourages us to compare ourselves with others. We see the wonderful things people do, and judge ourselves on how well we've done. All this can lead us to have negative thoughts about our world and ourselves. It becomes increasingly difficult for people to remain positive.

Perspective can control everything I just said. You have the power and ability to change the narrative. We are embarking on a quest to stop the simulation. The new path to success is right in front of you. You just need the right tools and knowledge to make it happen. You will live a happier and healthier lifestyle if you choose the path that you are currently on. It's filled with optimism and provides clarity.

This is not an easy trip, but it is beautiful. There is always resistance to anything worthwhile. It is the same principle that applies to a beginner guitarist. It is uncomfortable and sometimes even painful for a guitarist to first place their fingers across the fretboard. Because their fingers don't feel comfortable with the position they're in or the sensation of the strings, this is called "unaccustomed". It is not that the guitarist isn't a natural. But, they don't know how to adapt to this new experience. The guitar may experience a lot of strain and even calluses. The more experienced guitarists didn't let the discomfort stop them. Instead, they persevered. It was worth it. Their fingers became stronger, and playing the guitar became easier. There are many people who quit when they experience discomfort. These people don't get much attention because they weren't able to push through and achieve the goals they set. Those people can't play the guitar.

It takes time and effort to build up strength and get used to the changes happening in your body. This is true whether you're exercising or playing the guitar. To achieve your ultimate goal, you need patience and perseverance. If you're not able or willing to persevere through any difficulties and discomfort, it is impossible to achieve the desired results. It is necessary to accept some pain and discomfort in order to make a life-changing transformation. I am not trying to discourage you but to prepare you to face the challenges ahead. It may take some time for you to start seeing results, but it's well worth the effort. You'll be amazed at how quickly you see results. It will make you wonder why you didn't start sooner. It will encourage you to keep moving forward. The best thing about exercising is that you don't reach a goal. It is a continuous process of moving the goal posts, so you can keep moving forward. This is why I call it a journey and no destination. You will always be building upon the foundations and breaking down mental and physical barriers that you have established for yourself.

The goal is to regain control of your mind and body. It is common to allow external factors and people to influence and control our minds and bodies, even when it is not obvious. We will be able have mental clarity, which will allow us face whatever we do every day. We will be able mentally and physically strong to take on any challenges that come our way and not be scared or timid. It is a mental shift that allows you instead to focus on how you can win and not how you might fall. This is a part and parcel of our humanity and we can use it to help us become better and more powerful people.

Exercise has many benefits

Include exercise into your daily life. There are many benefits. There wouldn't have been any medical professionals recommending it. Although most of us are aware that exercising has physical benefits such as improving muscle size and heart health. However, there is more. Although the physical benefits are important and well-respected, they are not often discussed as much as the mental health benefits. It should.

Many people do not stick with their exercise routine because of its physical benefits. Instead, they do so because it brings them happiness and enhances their mood. This feeling is felt both while exercising and throughout the day. When something makes you feel good, people are more likely than ever to do it. This is where exercise shines. It's not the long-term advantages that matter. But it's the immediate benefits that will keep you going.

Exercise can have a tremendously positive effect on your mood. People who exercise feel happier, more energetic, as well as more positive. Exercise doesn't require you to be a gym rat to reap its benefits. It doesn't take much to see some benefits from moving more than you usually do. This makes it easy to exercise and improve your mental well-being.

It lowers your chances of having depression, anxiety, or negative moods

Studies on exercise and depression have been numerous and positive. Exercise can be used to treat mild-to-moderate depression with a similar efficacy rate to antidepressant medication. This allows people on medication to gradually reduce their dependence by increasing their exercise. It also has the added benefit of not having any side effects like medication. It is a clean and simple way to get rid of depression.

Harvard T.H. Chan School of Public Health. Researchers discovered that people who ran for 15 minutes each day or walked an hour per day had a 26% reduction in their risk of major depressive disorder (Robinson, et al. 2019, 2019). You can still reap the incredible benefits of this exercise even though it is not very much. Exercise has many effects on the brain that can help fight depression. These changes include new thought and feeling pathways that promote calmness and wellbeing as well as neural growth. Endorphins are chemicals which make you feel good, energized and happy. These endorphins are also released when we do something we enjoy, spend our time with those we love, and eat our favourite meals. These chemicals make you want come back for more because they make you feel good.

Exercise can help reduce anxiety and improve mood. Because exercise helps release tension and stress from the body. When you exercise, you must keep your eyes on the task at hand and only pay attention to it. This gives you a break from anxiety and negative emotions. Sometimes all that is needed is a little break. Exercise is the perfect example. Your exercise will make you feel positive and you won't be feeling deprived. If you ever feel anxious, or in a bad mood you can try to get out of your present environment and move around a little.

The positive effects can be felt almost immediately.

## Better Sleep

Negative moods and poor sleeping habits contribute to anxiety and depression. Because it is the time when our bodies heal themselves and reset, we need to go to bed. A refreshed mind is more capable of thinking clearly and can be in a better mood. You need to make sure you get enough sleep each night. It can be difficult to sleep well if this is the case.

People who exercise throughout the day often have better sleep quality at night. Do not exercise close to bedtime. It will make it harder for you to fall asleep. Endorphins and other chemicals released during exercise can give you an energy boost. But you don't need it when you're trying to go to sleep. It is best to exercise in the evening at least two hours before going to bed.

There are many theories on why exercise makes it easier to sleep well at night. One is that exercise is better for your brain. Many people wake up with racing thoughts. You will have a better night's sleep if you don't do this. It's clear that exercise can improve your sleep quality and help you fall asleep faster. Another theory is that you can wear your body out by exercising and cause it to strain. For your body to heal and reenergize itself after exercise, it needs to get enough sleep. You'll feel less tired and more comfortable falling asleep when it is time to go to bed. You can do it! See how you sleep better when you include a bit of exercise in your daily and/or weekly routines.

Helps manage stress

The hormone cortisol, which is released when you exercise, helps your body to deal with stress. This is the hormone that helps your body deal stress. You exercise and put your body under physical stress. This hormone helps your body deal with this stress. This hormone is good for your body and mind. You can calm down and release cortisol if you're under stress.

Exercise can give you something else to consider. When you exercise, it can be difficult to think about anything else. You can focus on your work if your mind gets distracted by the stressor. This will not just take your mind off of the stress but will also allow you to do a better workout.

## Chapter 7: Find a type of exercise that you like

Many people become stuck in doing exercises that seem too simple. You will find that when someone decides they want exercise, the first thing they do to stay active is enroll in the gym. While the gym is an excellent place to exercise, it may not work for everyone. Each person is unique and the exercise that works for them will not work for others. This is a journey to discover what works best for you and not to copy what others do.

The problem with exercise is that you can't keep up if your heart doesn't beat. When you are doing something you love, exercise is easier to sustain. It is important to find a form you are passionate about in order to make exercise a part of your daily routine. You have many options for getting your exercise in. This allows you to find the exercise that you love. When you truly enjoy the exercise, it will make it easier to stay consistent.

So, how do you choose the exercise you enjoy? There are so many to choose from that it can seem overwhelming. You also need to consider equipment or memberships for many types of exercise. Don't spend money on something you don't enjoy. It is important to take the time and narrow down your options in order to identify the best exercise. While you might need to try many different kinds of exercise to find the best one, it's much easier to narrow your choices.

Here are some questions you might ask yourself to determine what types of exercise you like best.

* Do you prefer being outdoors or in the indoors?

* Do you prefer to be with a small group of people or by myself?

* Would you be interested in taking up a sport?

* Do you want to do something fast or slow?

Answering these questions honestly will help you to find a good place to start. If you'd rather be outdoors, you might consider jogging, or cycling. You can also take a class with other people if you prefer to do your workouts in a small group. There are so many exercises to choose from that it is almost certain that you will find one that suits your needs.

It's important to find the right type of exercise for you and make time for it. This is how consistency is key to exercising and will help you see the best results. Once you have made a decision to do a certain exercise, it is important that you give it your all. After about a month, you can make your final decision. It is fine to keep it if your love for it. If not, it is OK to switch to something else.

You don't have the right type of exercise to follow for the rest your life. You can choose to vary it as much or little as necessary. This is a fantastic way to keep it new and to enjoy the exercise. If you're doing the same exercise and the same routine, it can be easy to get bored. Change it up to keep it interesting. You'll find you enjoy it more if there are changes you make. If you notice you are becoming bored, or you don't like it anymore, then it is time to make some changes. You can make a significant difference in your mood and experience by making a small adjustment.

I will be sending regular emails to all who wish to join me in my journey. I want this journey to be one that we can share together. These pages are designed to provide support for you in different aspects of your journey. These will have exercises, tips, tricks, motivational phrases, self-evaluation checks, self evaluation checklists, and success stories based on people who have been there. This is much more than a book. It is a journey that you want me to guide you. I truly care about you, your progress and how you feel. The book will contain more information on this as well as where you can sign-up.

Identifying your Why

It is the reason that will guide you on this journey. It will be the basic understanding of the reasons or reasons why you're doing what you are doing. If you understand why, you can overcome any barriers in your life that may be preventing you from reaching the full potential of your potential. The most powerful tool in your arsenal is your 'why'.

It's time you were honest with yourself

To truly understand why you're embarking on this journey, you must first be honest with your self. It's easy to give up on a basic reason for exercising. These reasons alone will not help you overcome any plateaus or mental blocks that might arise. You need a "why", which is grounded in something that you deeply believe in and desire to make this journey and your life a success.

You will need to spend some time searching for your 'why.' You won't wake up one day and realize your 'why. When you ask the right question and are willing to dig deeper into what you want, you will find it. Most people never do this. That's why so many people struggle to find meaning or purpose in their lives. This may seem like a lot to do for exercise but it can be done for any other area of your life.

Your "why" when it comes exercise will determine your motivation. It will also help you get motivated to exercise. Ask yourself these questions:

* Why would I like to improve my mental wellness?

* Why should I improve my mood

* Why would I like to move in a more forward direction?

It may prove to be more difficult for some than you might think. It may be something that you have known for a while, but didn't know how. Asking why is an excellent way to ensure you are reaching the root answer. Let's take as an example the first question. Let's take the first question as an example. The next step is to think about why you desire more self-esteem. You will likely answer "I want higher self-esteem" and "I want to feel more confident so that my thoughts can be controlled." Next, ask yourself why do you want to control your thoughts and your life. Next, you could say, "I want greater control over my thoughts, because I want take an active role in the lives of others, not be limited by negativity and obstacles."

You can keep going if you wish. You can reach your true purpose by finding the most profound version of your "why". Only you will be able to identify it once you find it. You should ask yourself why at the very least two to three times. This will allow you to dig down to the root of your "why". Many people believe they know what their 'why' is. Your 'why" would have been improving your mental wellbeing if you had read this book. This might sound like a good enough "why", but it's so vague you'd struggle to use it to motivate you when you need it. You must find the real reason behind your actions. This is why it's important to take your time, dig deep and go onward until you find the real reason for this journey. As you continue moving forward, you'll begin to realize how valuable this can be.

Your 'why?' does not have to be just one thing. It is possible to have many 'whys. In order to understand the root cause of something, you may need to ask many different kinds of questions. This stage of the journey focuses on self reflection and self-discovery. You will discover more about your self by doing this than you can from any other activity. This new journey will be more worthwhile if you get to the root of your desire.

You need to realize that your why' and goals are different. Your goals can be your why', but not your why'. Your why' is the ultimate goal. It is the end goal you aim for and what motivates you. Your goals are the things you wish to accomplish. Some of your goals might be to lose weight, feel more confident and more energetic. These are all possible short-term goals. While they may not be enough to keep you sane, these goals are still essential. I will be more specific about short-term goals later in this book. At the moment, we will just be focusing on our ultimate 'why'.

It can be hard to figure out your 'why'. This is because you are forced to confront your biggest problems. In essence, you are trying evaluate what you have put in your history. You are taking stock of what is holding your back and making the decision not to keep them there. You are also making decisions about your future and the steps you will take to get there. You won't reach the end of your journey because you will keep improving and pushing the goal line further. It doesn't mean you will never achieve your goals. It is the exact opposite. After you achieve your goals, you'll create new ones in order to keep moving forward.

Here are some examples to help you start thinking about yours.

* To conquer and manage anxiety so that each day can be more positive and fulfilling.

* For my children, so I can be more active and engaged with them.

* To search for love.

* To look and feel better about myself.

* To perform to an even higher standard at work.

* Give yourself more mental space and clarity to help you reach your career goals and move forward.

* For my family to be proud and instilled.

These could be the ones that appeal to you. They could also be used to help you dig deeper into yourself if that is what you want.

Motivation and Why It Is Important

Motivation can be a great motivator. It makes it possible to work hard and achieve our potential. Motivation can encourage us to take on the tough things that were holding us back in our past. Being able manage your motivation will allow you to take more control of your life.

Every decision you make is affected by your current motivation. If you have low motivation, you may choose not to do something. But if you have high motivation, you will be able and willing to do whatever it takes. This is what motivates. It's likely that you have experienced high and low levels of motivation. You'll see how much easier it can be to achieve something when you have your motivation behind you.

Motivated learners retain information faster and are better at learning. This is true no matter if you are studying to pass an exam or learning about a new exercise move. You are more productive and can concentrate better. Motivation is one powerful tool you can use to keep motivated. So, how do you stay motivated? Motivation can fluctuate, meaning that your motivation may be high at times and low at others. There are several things you can do to improve your motivation when you are feeling down.

Tap Into Your Curiosity

Curiosity can be a motivator as it pushes us to dig deeper and discover more. It stimulates us to move. The most curious people were the most successful. Because they believed there was greater potential, they sought out new and better ways to accomplish their goals. They believed there was more they could learn and more things to do. To be more motivated, you must get curious.

Exercise can be as simple as being curious. This will stimulate something inside of you and increase your motivation. You should also try new things if your current routine is getting boring.

## Chapter 8: Motivating People Surround You

You must surround yourself with the right people to keep you motivated. The people around you can have a significant impact on your ability to achieve your goals. This is because our subconsciously affects the people we surround us with. We are more likely than not to imitate positive, highly motivated people in our lives. You can look around your immediate circle to see who is most motivated and optimistic. Make an effort to spend more quality time with them and discuss your goals. This will allow them to hold you responsible if necessary. If you feel discouraged or unable to motivate yourself, you can talk to someone.

Your friends, family, and coworkers don't need to have the same goals. They just need to feel positive and motivated to achieve their dreams. This energy will fuel your growth. It feels great to share your accomplishments, with people you trust will support them. This will help you feel motivated and can be a great way to let others know how far you've come.

Learn more about those who have reached their goals.

It is extremely motivating to learn about the successes of others. They don't necessarily have to have the same goals as yours to be inspiring. You can read about successful business people, activists, athletes and other individuals who have accomplished great things or achieved a huge goal. You'll feel inspired by it and want to do more.

The other benefit of doing this is the fact that you're constantly learning. You might also learn new techniques and tips on how to stay motivated, or achieve your goals. A lot can be learned from people with lots of experience. If you're feeling down or unmotivated, a biography or autobiography may be the perfect thing to help you get back on track. The idea is not to try to emulate the lives of others, but to draw inspiration from their stories to help us on our own personal journeys.

Do it Now

Analytical paralysis is an illness. Analyzing paralysis occurs when you spend too much time planning, reviewing and thinking about something, that you don't have the motivation or energy to actually do it. It's almost like telling yourself to stop doing something. We will talk more about planning later. But, everything doesn't have to be perfect before it is time to get started. It doesn't hurt to have a plan in place from the beginning.

You will learn more about how it works and make improvements as you go along.

I like the analogy of riding on a bicycle. If you're on a bicycle and are pedaling, the handlebars can be moved in any direction you wish. But if you don't move and just sit on your bicycle, it won't be possible to turn the handlebars in the direction you want. You won't get anywhere, and your efforts to direct yourself will not pay off. This is why you need to get moving. Planning is essential, but it must not be overshadowed by actual movement. You can set a time limit on your planning. This will keep you from over-planning and help you set a goal for when to get started.

Intuitively re-examine your Why and become a part of it

This chapter focused on finding your "why" and making sure it is at the forefront in everything you do. You can decide whether to share it with others and wear the badge of honour, or keep it for yourself and use as a silent obstacle remover. It is vital that your 'why' is internalized so that you can refer to it whenever you need. Your 'why?' will be your greatest motivational tool. It's easy to return to when you need motivation.

Keep your 'why?' in your head. It is possible to do this by fully immersing your self in it. Set reminders to your phone so that a message pops up. Put it on sticky note and place them where you will see them. Every morning, take some time to reflect on your "why". All these things will help to keep your "why" in mind. This will keep you inspired and show you why this is the journey you want.

If you reach this point in your book, but still have not found your why', it is time to really dig into yourself and do some soul searching. It's up to you to decide what works for you. However, it's important to be open to the challenge of finding your 'why. Discover what motivates and inspires you. This will help you keep going even when it's difficult. Your 'why" is the most powerful tool for motivation you will ever find.

3

Make Your First Step a Success

The hardest step in any new journey is usually the first. This is not because the first step is the most difficult, but because of its mental aspect. The first step is a radical change from your usual routine. This means that you're asking your self to do something entirely different. Our brains and bodies prefer the familiar. When we do something new, it means that we are stepping into something unfamiliar. This can make the first step toward success difficult. It is possible to overcome these obstacles and get on with the next step.

Even the greatest people have started somewhere. It is important to remember that small steps lead to great results. It is all about getting started. Once you've taken the first step, everything will become easier. This is because momentum can propel you forward. It's easier to keep moving if you're already moving. It's possible to get your mind and body ready and enjoy the joy of big changes.

Get started with mental preparation

Preparing for the first step is key to success. Because your mind holds you back, this is why it is important to prepare. By breaking down mental barriers, your mind will allow you to do more and be open to the possibility that you might have to do difficult things. This can be done whenever you want to exercise. Each time, there are new mental barriers. You will have days where you just don't feel like working out. These are the days you need to be more reliant on your mental preparedness. It is possible to overcome this if you do the right thing. Mental preparation helps you manage stress levels and decrease fears. Mentally and physically well-prepared people will be better prepared for anything.

Remind yourself of your "Why"

You should always remember your "why". This is the thing that will keep your going even when you feel discouraged. It can be difficult to break through and move, but understanding why you do it will help break down any mental barriers. This can be described as taking out your sword and getting ready for battle.

It might be worth writing down your "why" on a note and putting it in your workout clothes or bag for gym. By writing down your 'why' on a note, you can see it when you go to get dressed and will be more prepared. It is possible to set up a phone reminder that will display the phrase at the time of your exercise. This will be not only a reminder you have to exercise but also remind you of why you are doing it.

Invent a Ritual

I discussed the fact our brains and bodies like familiarity. You can actually use this to your advantage if you are mentally preparing for something. These are routines that you repeat over and over. They're easy to remember and can help you achieve the results that you desire. Start with a routine to make things easier.

This routine or ritual will make you unique. It is important to choose something that you enjoy and that puts you in the right mindset for what lies ahead. Numerous celebrities and sports figures have a routine or ritual that they follow before they take to the stage. This helps them relax and find their comfort. The All Blacks New Zealand Rugby team performs the Haka before every match. Michael Jordan used college shorts underneath his current team's. These are just some of the many rituals we are familiar with, but there are probably many more that people don't want to share. While it might sound strange, this ritual works for me. I rinse my hands with cold water and wait for the next 30 seconds before starting any exercise. This is like a trigger for my brain and helps me get in the zone. My mind knows when it's time for it to happen.

These rituals may be useful as a starting point. But the best ones are those that you create. It might take some time before you find what works best for your needs. Test out several rituals until you find one that gives you the energy and motivation to get through the day. Because this will be your personal ritual, you are free to be as imaginative as you wish.

## Feel the thrill of conquering your first steps

If you've ever overcome a fear or achieved a big goal, you will know how great it feels. Even if it's not something you've done, you will soon feel that feeling once you finish this book. It's an amazing feeling. Sometimes you just stand there in amazement and wonder for a while. It is because you achieved something you had always wanted. You have overcame all the physical and mental barriers that you had faced.

This feeling is caused by the fact that you believe you have what it takes to achieve your goal. There will be times in any difficult journey when it is easy to think that you might not have the ability to reach your goal. This has happened to me, and you have got to get over it. As a way of stopping those thoughts taking control, you can use your 'why. When you conquer the first step, it gives you the confidence to go on. This provides an additional boost of motivation that will help you keep going. This will be something you'll always be able to look back at and prove to yourself that you are capable of completing the first step. The hardest step is the first, but that doesn't mean you can't do anything else. This feeling is something you will be able to hold onto for life. This is another tool you can use to battle doubts and insecurities when they occur.

Exercise is great to your physical and psychological health. It boosts endorphins and makes you feel happy. For your overall health, movement and exercise are so important. You can reap huge benefits by simply moving around every hour, or even taking a walk during lunch. Don't feel defeated by the task before you. Give yourself something to look forward. If you want to be excited about something, then you will need to conquer the obstacle in your path. Use these strategies to overcome your first obstacle and experience that great feeling at the end. You will soon see that it is its own reward. And as you keep going, it will become more enjoyable.

Performance Anxiety

It's quite common for people to suffer from performance anxiety. Although performance anxiety is most commonly referred to by athletes, it's not something that happens only to professionals. Performance anxiety can happen to anyone who is faced with a challenge. Many people think that exercise is a matter of how they feel physically. This is not true. Mental blocks are common and can affect how you feel when you're exercising. Some people feel unworthy or too hard. These thoughts are very common, but it doesn't mean they are true. It means that you're not the only one feeling this way, and that there are many options to help you counter it.

Get It

If you are experiencing this, you must catch it immediately. You may find excuses or negative comments about your fitness. These are indicators that can be picked up. At this point, you can get back control over your mind. If you don't recognize it right away, your mind may run wild and you might decide to skip the exercise.

These negative thoughts can manifest in physical sensations. This could be the cause of butterflies in the stomach or tightening the muscles. It can also lead to faster heart rate. It is important to stop thinking before you do. Reflect on the times you have been able to accomplish difficult tasks and the feelings you had when you finished them. Find your 'why,' and use it as inspiration. Anything that distracts you from the negative thoughts and keeps your mind clear will be of benefit to you.

The Challenge is yours

You are experiencing your body's natural stress responses. There are two options your body may be trying to tell you. These are your flight or fight reflexes. You can choose to either fight the anxiety and get the benefit of the exercise, or avoid it completely so you don't have to deal anymore with the feelings. Either of these options will help you to calm down your anxiety. However, one option will bring about a positive outcome while the other one will only cause you to feel neutral. You know your ultimate goal so it's best to just keep fighting.

You can control your mind. It's not reversed. You can beat it, even though it may feel uncomfortable for a time. You are investing for a better future. To get there, you have got to step out of your comfort zones. It might be nice to live in comfort, but there are no plants or animals that thrive and grow in it. Everything that grows must overcome challenges to be the best version of itself. For babies to grow and develop, they must endure teething and growing pains. This is part of daily life. It may not always be easy but it is well worth the effort.

Calm your Body and Mind

Sometimes, all you really need is calm. Performance anxiety can make it hard to think clearly and execute your actions appropriately. This is when your body goes into fight/flight mode. In many cases, the flight side of things prevails. In such cases, it is best to step away from the situation for a while and to take some time to breath. It may sound simple but breathing can calm you and give your brain some much-needed oxygen.

The goal of breathing is calm your body. In doing so, you'll notice a calmer mind. Deep breathing is a great way to relax your muscles and slow down your heart beat. It is best to concentrate on your breathing. Pay attention to how much time and how deeply you are breathing. You can take the time to focus on the rise or fall of your chest. This awareness will help you to forget everything else. This will help to focus on what is most important. When you feel calm, you'll find it much easier for you to give up and try again.

It will be the most difficult step on your journey, but it will be one of the most valuable. You will find that it will propel you forward. You will reach goals and achieve highlights you never imagined possible. This is just the beginning of building the foundation. Once you get there, you will be able to handle it and make this a permanent part of you life.

## Chapter 9: Attainable Goals

It is one of the best ways to help you reach your ultimate goal. Knowing where you want to go, you now need a plan. The steps that lead to your ultimate goal are the goals I am referring to.

Each small step can be taken one at a time until you reach the ultimate goal. As you work towards each goal, you'll find yourself more motivated. It's almost addictive. This feeling of success captures you and makes you eager to take the next step. It will be clear that many of your limitations are just illusions and can be overcome. Each small victory will make the process much more enjoyable. Finding something you enjoy doing is the best way to make progress. This is because you can set your goals in the right manner.

How to Set Goals

Tony Robbins was a motivational speaker who is also a philanthropist and is well-known for his powerful words. I will be referring to them throughout this chapter. To make your goals a reality, you need to set goals.

But, setting goals is crucial. But how can you do this? This is a great question. It will help guide you in finding the perfect way of setting goals. There's a right and a wrong way of setting goals. Failure to do so will result in frustration and unmet goals. If you do things the right way, you'll reap the benefits and enjoy the whole process more.

Set Smart Goals

This is one rule that you should follow when you set goals. This will allow you to set realistic goals and make you feel accomplished. I will show you how to use

SMART goals in your goal setting. SMART stands in for the following:

S-pecific

The first letter stands to indicate specific. That means any goal you establish should be clear and concise. Setting goals can be tempting. Many people don't take the time and put in the effort to be specific when setting goals. This can lead to two things: either the goal is too far away or it doesn't have a clear end. One example is that you decide to improve your friendship with a friend. It sounds great but it is not clear how to achieve this goal. A goal is meant to guide you in your actions.

This broad goal could be your starting point. You will need to be more specific if you wish to improve your friendship. This would mean that you should call your friend every week to check in on them and to catch up. This is something you should do. It's a useful goal, as it is specific and will help you know what to do.

M-easurable

It is important to have a measurable goal. A measurable objective will have a number that shows how far you are away from the goal. You can use dates, time, amounts, or any other form of numeric measurement to indicate your progress towards the goal. This will allow to you see the extent of your success as you work towards your goal. You can see the measurements in the example. Your friend must be contacted once a week. This tells you how often and how many times you should call. These measurements will be required to achieve your goal.

For a better understanding of the concept, you could also use it in the context of exercise. If you are just starting to exercise and would like to increase your running distance, time spent running, and steps taken if you have an electronic pedometer, this could be your goal. This will allow to you measure how far you are from your goal. It will also help to monitor your progress. For example, in the first week you could set your goal for 10 minutes. Next week, you might add an additional two minutes. This will allow for you to improve. If you find 10 minutes too long, you can decrease the amount to 5 mins. You can easily adjust the goals to make improvements.

A-ttainable

The temptation to simply use your goal as a starting goal is a big one when setting goals. Our abilities are usually greater when we begin the task than they are once we have completed it. This is why people often give up halfway through the challenge and go back to the drawing board after a few weeks. Unrealistic goals can have the opposite effect. You might feel demoralized and want to quit, as the goal seems impossible. It is important to avoid it at all costs.

To set goals, it is essential to first know your current situation. A trial might be a good idea for exercising. This will allow you to assess your current fitness level and help you to set realistic goals. Spend some time lifting weights, cardio, or doing whatever exercise regimen you plan to use. See how far you can go before you become tired. This will help you set your goals.

It is important to not set unrealistic goals. It will not be rewarding to complete goals that require little effort. If you look at your trial, you may have found that you were able do 10 pushups before stopping. It would be impossible to reach 50 pushups with your current strength. However if you aim for just 10 pushups, you won't be challenging yourself. The ideal goal is 15 to 20 pushups. Although it may be challenging it is also achievable. It's possible to push yourself a bit more than you think when you exercise.

Relevant

It is important that your goals are related to the life you desire. It is important that all of the small goals you set lead to your ultimate goal. Every situation is different, so don't compare your goals to others. A person might set a goal to go to sleep earlier in order to have more time for their projects. However, this might not work for them because they need to get out of bed early to exercise. Set your goals in the context of where and when you want them to lead.

Time Bound

You must set a deadline for any goal that you have. It can be easy to let it drag on for ever if it doesn't. If there is a deadline, we are more motivated to achieve our goals. A deadline or time frame is more motivating than not having one. This will make it easier to think we can do everything we want, and to stop taking action when necessary. Things that have a deadline will always be the priority in our life.

It is possible that a student will not study enough for an exam if they have limited time. It's not because the material is difficult or too hard, it's just that people tend to procrastinate on things that have no deadline. This is natural, but it must be managed to ensure that things can be done in a timely manner. When you can set a time limit for the task, you will be more motivated.

You need to set realistic goals and allow yourself enough time to reach them. It is important to evaluate what you want and what your life looks at this time, then make a decision regarding the timeframe. As you work towards your goals, you will be able to determine how long you must spend to reach them. Start by setting goals and then adjust your timeline if necessary.

Write down your goals

Another tip for setting goals is writing them down. Although it might be tempting just to keep your goal in your head for now, writing them down will help you make them concrete. They become tangible and real. It is almost like writing a contract with yourself. It is much less likely that you will forget about what you have written. Even if you lose the paper, writing is a way to embed it in your brain. This is why taking notes during seminars and lectures is important. Even if it's not necessary to go back and review the notes, taking notes will help you retain the information better because you are actively learning.

It is important to take the time and write down your goals. The words "I would prefer to", "hopefully", and/or "might" are not strong enough for you to believe that it is possible. Instead, speak with the words "I'll" or "I Can." This will create a belief in yourself that you can accomplish your goals. It is almost as if you have no other choice. This is motivating.

Once you have written out your goals, it is important that you are able see them. You can place them anywhere you know you'll see them. Place notes about your goals in places that are not tempting to abandon them. For example, if your goal to eat healthier in order to fuel your workouts better, you could place a note in your fridge or in your kitchen cabinet. If you open the doors, the reminder will always be there so you are more likely to follow through with your goal. Place the reminder where you can see it.

Here are some layouts for goal setting that I designed. You can draw inspiration from this layout and alter it to your liking. The most important thing to remember is to keep track of your progress. You also need a place where you can record notes about how the workout went. This will enable you to keep track of your progress and provide a way to see how you felt about your mental health.

This is an example of running:

My Goals - Running - 1st Jan 2021

WHY? (Insert There)

Goal - Distance Time Frame

Run 1km (non stop) - 1km - 14th Jan 2021

Note to self - Slow it down. Always warm up and stretch properly. Take the time to work towards your goal. You can do it every other morning, at 07:30 AM. This is possible.

Run 2.5km (non stop) - 2.5km - 1st Feb 2021

Notes to self: I achieved the 1k goal. Already confident in my final goal. I have had a few issues with my start times and hiccups but these will be fixed. It is important to note how positive I feel mental after a run. That's what I want all the times.

Run 4km (non stop) - 4km - 1st March 2021

Notes to myself - Reached the 2.5k goal. It felt difficult, sometimes felt heavy. I know I can do this 4k.

Run 6km (non stop) - 6km - 1st April 2021

Notes for self - I did it! It's incredible that I can get this far. I never thought that it was possible. You should also continue to map your runs every night. It's easier to run if you're not distracted by my destination.

Run 7.5km (non stop) - 7.5km - 1st May 2021

Notes to Self - 6k was my goal, and I'm proud. Although I was slower than expected, I'm making good progress. To make up for the lost goal, I plan to run five times per week. I'm proud of my achievements but I refuse miss another goal.

Run 10km (non stop) - 10km - 1st June 2021

Notes to Self - 7.5k complete and in great times! A month more to hit the 10k, and I feel super confident based upon the past month of progress. I feel so much better and there is no stopping me.

1st June 2021

10km run completed.

Let's look at an example to help you lose weight.

My Goals – Weight Loss (225lbs), 1st Jan 2021

The Road to $200

WHY? (Insert There)

Goal – Current Weight - Timeframe

220lbs to 225lbs - 1st february 2021

Notes to yourself - This goal is achievable. Keep to your workout schedule and be consistent with your food intake. You can do it. Remember why this is important. Be sure to keep track of any roadblocks. Anything you have ever struggled with. It will help to overcome them.

215 - 219 Pounds - 1st of March 2021

Notes to myself - I reached my goal of 219 lbs. This is a remarkable progression. Running becomes less common, and lifting weights feels easier. Feeling happy both mentally & physically and eager to improve. Keep breaking down those barriers.

210lbs – 213lbs – 1st April 2020

Notes for self - Reached goal (213 lbs weigh in) I'm amazed at how great it feels! It is now a routine that I love and it's becoming a way of life. I feel so relaxed mentally. I feel so optimistic about my future.

205lbs – 207lbs – 1st May 2021

Notes to myself - I reached my goal of 207 lbs. Running has improved so much, although I'm not so good at weight training. I managed to run my first 10k. Love my new self. I feel better than ever in a long while.

200lbs - 202lbs - 1st June 2021

Notes for self: I couldn't feel more proud of myself. I feel like a different person. The journey doesn't stop there. I have a set of new goals that I want to achieve in the next six months.

1st June 2021

Final weight in - 193 lbs

Action Your Goals

Setting goals is a good idea. Make sure you have an action program to help you reach them. It's easy to set your goals and not develop an action program. Every goal does not have all the steps. One example is to lose a pound each week. This is a very SMART goal. However, there must be more to it in order to reach your goal. It is important to create an action plan.

A good plan would be to get rid of junk food and candy. Next, it's time to visit the grocery store to buy healthy and low-calorie foods. Another option is to go for a walk each day after dinner. All these steps together will help you reach your goal. It's a step-by-step guide that explains exactly what you should do in order reach your goal. It is a good idea to look at your goals in order to determine if you can break them up into smaller steps. This will help you work more efficiently towards your goals.

www.ingramcontent.com/pod-product-compliance
Lightning Source LLC
Chambersburg PA
CBHW050406120526
44590CB00015B/1846